The Definitive Dash Diet Guidebook for Busy People

Don't Waste Your Time and Get Back in Shape with Amazing and Super Affordable Recipes

Demi Cooper

Table of contents

Salmon and Cucumber Platter

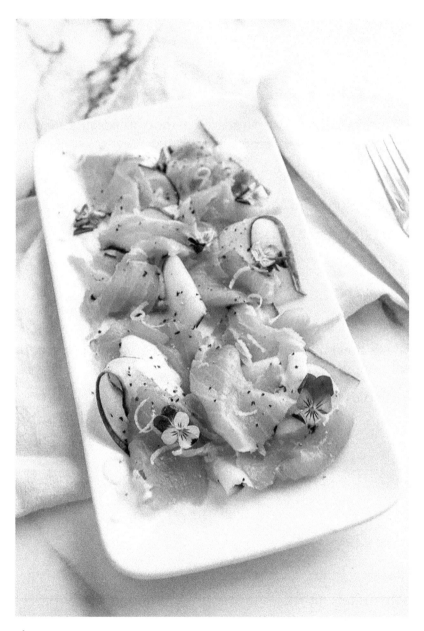

Serving: 4

Prep Time: 10 minutes

Cook Time: nil

Ingredients:

- 2 cucumbers, cubed
- 2 teaspoons fresh squeezed lemon juice ounces non-fat yogurt teaspoon lemon zest, grated
- Pepper to taste
- teaspoons dill, chopped
- 8 ounces smoked salmon, flaked

How To:

1. Take a bowl and add cucumbers, juice , lemon peel , pepper, dill,salmon, yogurt and toss well.

2.   Serve cold.

3.   Enjoy!

Nutrition (Per Serving)

Calories: 242

Fat: 3g

Carbohydrates: 3g

Protein: 3g

Tuna Paté

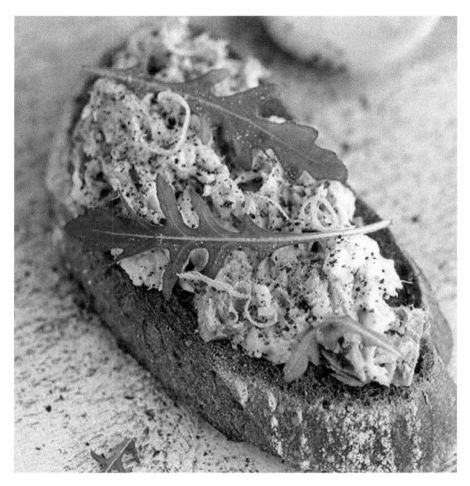

Serving: 4

Prep Time: 10 minutes

Cook Time: nil

Ingredients:

- ounces canned tuna, drained and flaked
- teaspoons fresh lemon juice 1 teaspoon onion, minced
- ounces low-fat cream cheese
- ¼ cup parsley, chopped

How To:

1.   Take a bowl and blend in tuna, cheese , juice , parsley, onion and stir well.

2.   Serve cold and enjoy!

Nutrition (Per Serving)

Calories: 172

Fat: 2g

Carbohydrates: 8g

Protein: 4g

Cinnamon Salmon

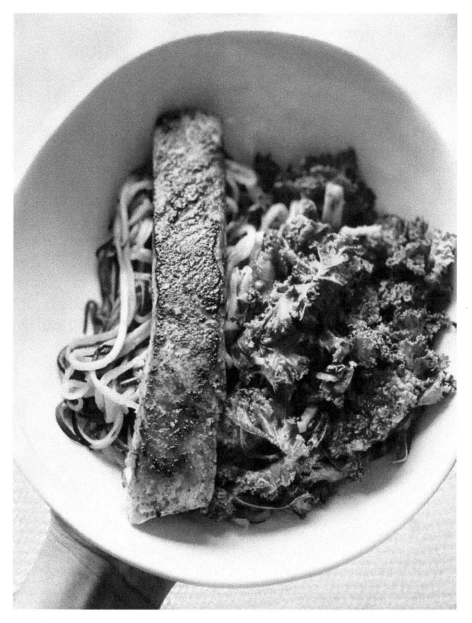

Serving: 4

Prep Time: 10 minutes

Cook Time: 10 minutes

Ingredients:

- 2 salmon fillets, boneless and skin on
- Pepper to taste
- 1 tablespoon cinnamon powder
- 1 tablespoon organic olive oil

How To:

1.   Take a pan and place it over medium heat, add oil and let it heat up.

2.   Add pepper, cinnamon and stir.

3.   Add salmon, skin side up and cook for five minutes on each side .

4.   Divide between plates and serve.

5.   Enjoy!

Nutrition (Per Serving)

Calories: 220

Fat: 8g

Carbohydrates: 11g

Protein: 8g

Chicken Bruschetta

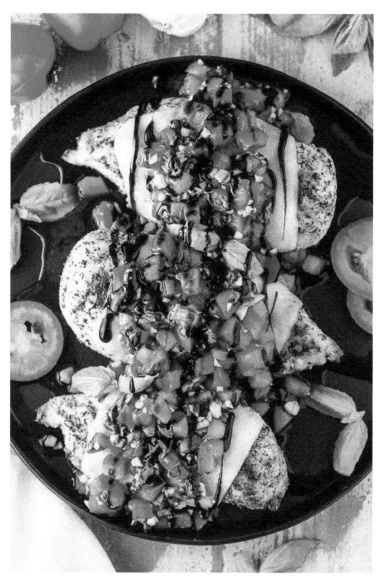

SmartPoints value: Green plan - 1SP, Blue plan - 1SP, Purple plan - 1SP

Total Time: 20 min, Prep time: 10 min, Cooking time: 10 min, Serves: 4

Nutritional value: Calories - 187, Carbs – 4.4g, Fat - 7g, Protein – 27.3g

When the weather is heating up, I mostly crave for fresh and light meals other than rich and comforting.

My most recently found new love when it comes to dessert is this deliciously prepared Italian Chicken Bruschetta. It's just so simple, simply made with

fresh tomatoes, basil, and garlic. I've tried it several times, and one sweet thing about it is the refreshing flavors. There is just something about the way the fresh and juicy tomato works together with the bright basil and bold garlic.

While preparing, I like to add some grilled chicken breast to it as a lean protein. If you've noticed, I do more of chicken breast, yes, because it is low in points, and it's a perfect way of adding protein to my meal without getting over budget with my points.

Ingredients

- Chicken breast (skinless, boneless) - 1 lb
- Large Roma tomatoes (finely diced) - 2 pieces
- Basil (finely chopped, fresh) - 1/4 cup
- Garlic (minced) - 2 cloves

- Olive oil (1 tbsp plus 1 tsp)

- Balsamic Vinegar (1/2 tsp)

- Parsley (dried) - 1 tsp

- Oregano (dried) - 1 tsp

- Pepper and Salt to taste

Instructions

1.   After cutting the chicken breasts into four equal-sized fillets, season each of the side of the chicken with the parsley, oregano and salt and pepper.

2.   Over medium-high heat, heat one teaspoon of olive oil in a medium-sized, nonstick skillet. For 4-5 minutes, cook as you turn each side until the chicken is entirely cooked and browned.

3.   Remove from heat and cover with a lid to allow it to sit for about 5 minutes.

4.   Make bruschetta by mixing tomatoes, olive oil, garlic, basil, balsamic vinegar, and pepper and salt in a bowl.

5.   Put the chicken breast on a plate and top each of them with about ¼ cup of the bruschetta. Then drizzle on some extra balsamic if you so desire.

6.   You can also make a sandwich with fresh Italian bread and little creamy goat cheese. The flavor is so bold and mouthwatering.

Lemon Chicken with Broccoli

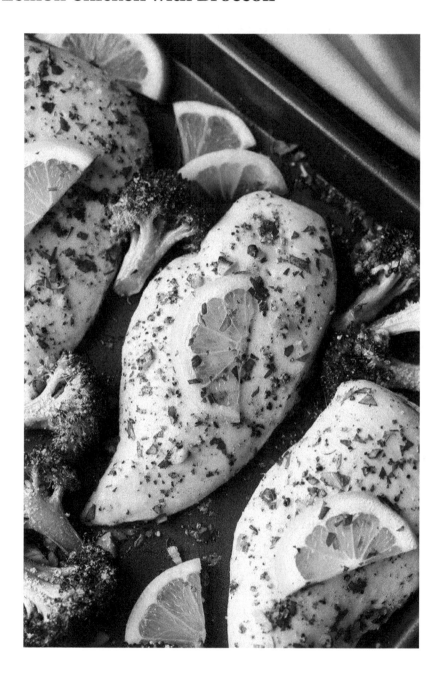

SmartPoints value: Green plan - 3SP, Blue plan - 1SP, Purple plan - 1SP

Total Time: 30 min, Prep time: 15 min, Cooking time: 15 min, Serves: 4

Nutritional value:

Calories - 176.6, Carbs - 8.4g, Fat - 2.0g, Protein - 32.3g

The whole family will love this fantastic weeknight dinner, and it's ready in just 30 minutes. To ensure that the chicken cooks quickly and evenly, you should slice it thinly. Cover the pan when cooking the broccoli to help build up steam, bathing the florets with heat. It will allow tops that aren't in contact with the hot pan to cook properly. You will need one small to medium head of broccoli to get enough florets and one lemon to yield enough zest and juice for this entrée.

Ingredients

- All-purpose flour - 2 Tbsp
- Black pepper - ¼ tsp (freshly ground)
- Fat-free, reduced-sodium chicken broth - 1½ cup(s) (divided)
- Fresh lemon juice - 1 Tbsp
- Fresh parsley - 2 Tbsp (chopped)
- Lemon zest - 2 tsp, or more to taste*

- Minced Garlic - 2 tsp
- Olive oil - 2 tsp
- Table salt - ½ tsp (divided)
- Uncooked chicken breast(s) -12 oz, thinly sliced (boneless, skinless)
- Uncooked broccoli - 2½ cup(s), small florets Instructions

Direction:

1.   On a clean plate, mix 1 1/2 Tbsp of flour, 1/4 tsp of salt, and pepper, then add chicken and turn to coat.

2.   Put a large nonstick skillet over medium-high heat and pour the oil in for heating.

3.   Add the chicken and cook, turning as needed, until it is lightly browned and cooked through, about 5 minutes; remove to a plate.

4.   Put one cup of broth and Garlic in the same skillet, then boil over high heat, scraping up browned bits from the bottom of the pan with a wooden spoon.

5.   Add the broccoli, then cover and cook for 1 minute.

6.   Stir the remaining 1/2 cup broth, 1/2 Tbsp flour, and 1/4 tsp salt together in a small cup, then add to the skillet and bring its content to a simmer over low heat.

7.   Cover the skillet and cook until the broccoli is crisp-tender and the sauce thickens slightly.

8.   Stir in the chicken and lemon zest, then heat through.

9.   Remove the skillet from heat, and stir in the parsley and lemon juice, then toss to coat.

Chicken and Fennel in Rosemary-wine Broth

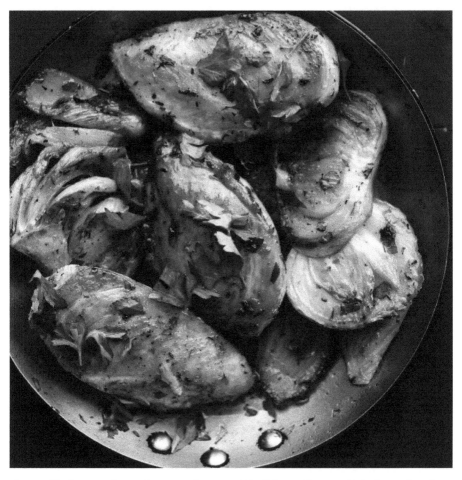

SmartPoints value: Green plan - 4SP, Blue plan - 2SP, Purple plan - 2SP

Total Time: 40 min, Prep time: 18 min, Cooking time: 22 min, Serves: 4

Nutritional value: Calories - 121.5, Carbs - 10.5g, Fat - 6.3g, Protein - 26.0g

If you are looking for a dish that will tickle your belly on a chilly night, this rustic Italian entrée is perfect, and since you will cook it in one skillet, that makes it easy to fix in your vegetable. You should first sear the chicken to produce an excellent brown exterior. You can then sauté the fennel and onion in the flavorful drippings left in the skillet. They will mix and become sweetened as they cook.

Return the chicken and any accumulated juices to the skillet to finish cooking.

Ingredients

- All-purpose flour - 5 tsp (divided)
- Black pepper - ⅛ tsp, or to taste (freshly ground)
- Canned chicken broth - 14½ oz
- Minced Garlic - 2 tsp
- Olive oil - 1 Tbsp, extra-virgin (divided)
- Red/white wine - 1/4 cup
- Rosemary - 1¼ tsp, fresh (chopped)
- Table salt - ½ tsp, or to taste
- Uncooked chicken breast(s) - 1 pound(s), cut into bite-size chunks (boneless, skinless)
- Uncooked fennel bulb(s) - 1 pound(s)
- Uncooked red onion(s) - 1 small (chopped)

Instructions

1.   Trim the stalk from fennel to quarter bulb(s) lengthwise and then slice in a cross-like manner into small pieces. Reserve the fronds for garnish (about 3 cups fennel will be available).

2.   Put the chicken on a plate and sprinkle it with rosemary, then sprinkle it with 4 tsp flour and toss to coat.

3.   Add 1 tsp of oil to a large nonstick skillet and heat over medium-high heat.

4.   Add the chicken and cook, occasionally turning with tongs, until it is lightly brown.

5.   Transfer the chicken to a clean plate (cooking is partial at this point).

6.   Heat the remaining 2 tsp oil in the same skillet over medium-high heat and add fennel and onion; sauté until it becomes lightly brown and almost tender.

7.   Add wine and Garlic, then reduce the heat to low and simmer, stirring the bottom of the pan to scrape up browned bits, until most of the wine has evaporated.

8.   Stir the broth together with the remaining 1 tsp flour in a small bowl and then stir into skillet.

9.   Add salt and pepper, then increase the heat to high and bring it to a boil. Reduce the heat to medium-low and simmer for another 1 minute.

10.   Add the chicken and cook, often tossing until the chicken cooks through. Garnish with reserved chopped fennel fronds and serve.

You can serve it with crusty whole-grain bread, or over rice, to mop up all of the broth.

If you prefer not to use wine in this recipe, you can substitute with one tablespoon of red or white wine vinegar and three tablespoons of water.

Chicken Cordon Bleu

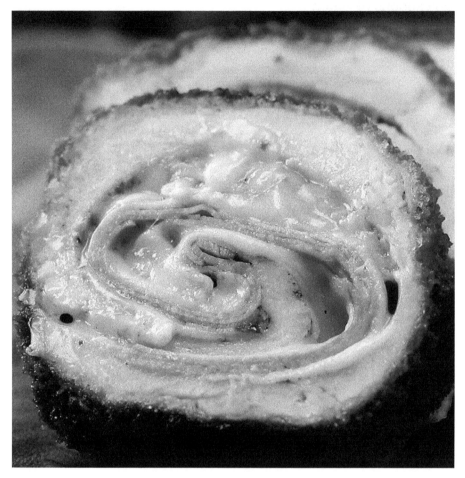

SmartPoints value: Green plan - 6SP, Blue plan - 4SP, Purple plan - 4SP

Total Time: 46 min, Prep time: 11 min, Cooking time: 35 min, Serves: 4

Nutritional value: Calories - 357.9, Carbs - 12.7g, Fat - 16.9g, Protein - 36.7g

Cordon bleu was a commonly served dish at dinner-parties in the sixties. Preparing it is simple: You sandwich a layer of ham and cheese between thin medallions of chicken or veal, then you sauté it.

Here, I have created a light version of the recipe to use a single layer of chicken rolled around the filling to make an elegant presentation.

Prepare this dish the next time you have guests and add some greens to the plate: either roasted broccolini, asparagus, or haricot vert (thin French green beans) will do just fine.

Ingredients

- All-purpose flour - 4 Tbsp
- Black pepper - ⅛ tsp (or to taste), freshly ground
- Cornflake crumbs - ½ cup(s)
- Lean ham (cooked) - 4 slice(s), (about 2 oz. total)
- Egg(s) - 1 large, lightly beaten
- Ground nutmeg - ⅛ tsp
- Parmesan cheese - 2 Tbsp, freshly grated
- Reduced-sodium chicken broth - ½ cup(s)
- Swiss cheese - 2 oz (4 thin slices), low-fat
- Table salt - ½ tsp
- Table wine - 1 Tbsp, Madeira

- Uncooked chicken breast(s) -1 pound(s), (4 breasts, 1/4 pound each), pounded to ¼-inch thickness (boneless, skinless)

- 2% reduced-fat milk - ½ cup(s)

Instructions

1.   Spray a baking sheet with nonstick spray while you preheat the oven to 400°F.

2.   Place one half of a chicken breast on a work surface and top it with one slice of the ham, then one slice of the Swiss cheese.

3.   Roll it up in a jelly-roll style, and secure with a toothpick. Repeat the process with the remaining chicken, ham, and cheese.

4.   Make a mixture of two tablespoons of flour, one-quarter teaspoon of salt, and ground pepper on a sheet of wax paper.

5.   Place the egg and the cornflake crumbs in separate shallow bowls.

6.   Taking it one at a time, coat the chicken rolls lightly, first with the flour mixture, and then dip it into the egg for a single layer coat.

7.   Coat the rolls with the cornflake crumbs, and place them on the baking sheet (discard any leftover flour mixture, egg, and cornflake bits).

8.   Spray the chicken rolls lightly with nonstick spray. Bake until the temperature of the rolls reaches 160°F, 30−35 minutes.

9.   To prepare the sauce, mix the milk, the broth, the Madeira, nutmeg, the remaining two tablespoons of flour, the remaining 1/4 teaspoon of salt, and another grinding of the pepper in a medium-sized saucepan.

10.   Whisk until it is smooth and cook over medium heat, continually whisking until it becomes thick in about 6 minutes.

11.   Remove the sauce from the heat and stir in the Parmesan cheese, then cover to keep it warm.

12.   When the chicken rolls are ready, drizzle them with the sauce and serve them immediately.

Southern-Style Oven-Fried Chicken

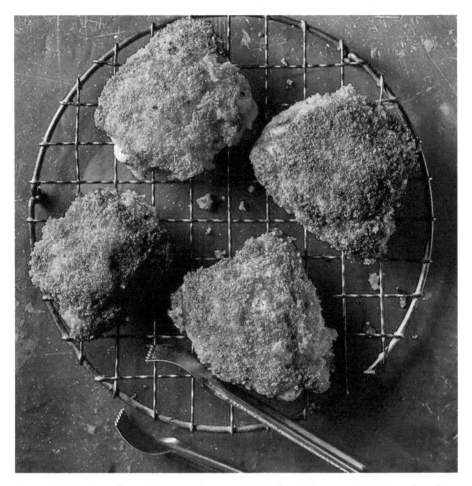

SmartPoints value: Green plan - 4SP, Blue Plan - 3SP, Purple plan - 3SP

Total Time: 45 min, Prep time: 15 min, Cooking time: 30 min, Serves: 4

Nutritional value: Calories - 256.9, Carbs - 31.3g, Fat - 1.6g, Protein - 27.5g

Switch to oven frying and lighten up this favorite hearty dish. I decided to improve the flavor by adding buttermilk and a pinch of cayenne pepper.

Ingredients

- All-purpose flour - ⅓ cup(s)
- Buttermilk (low-fat) - 3 oz
- Cayenne pepper - ¼ tsp (or to taste), divided
- Cooking spray - 3 spray(s)
- Cornflake crumbs - ½ cup(s)
- Table salt - ½ tsp (or to taste), divided
- Uncooked chicken breast(s) - 1 pound(s), four 4-oz pieces (boneless, skinless)

Instructions

1.   Heat the oven to 375°F before starting. Coat a 13- X 8- X 2-inch baking dish lightly with cooking spray and set it aside.

2.   Add salt and cayenne pepper to chicken for a tasty seasoning and set it aside also.

3.   Put a mixture of flour, 1/4 teaspoon salt, and 1/8 teaspoon cayenne pepper in a bowl of medium size.

4.   Put the buttermilk and cornflakes crumbs in 2 separate shallow bowls.

5. Dip the chicken in the flour mixture and evenly coat both sides.

6. Next, dip the flour-coated chicken into buttermilk and turn it to coat both sides.

7. Finally, dip the coated chicken in cornflake crumbs and turn to coat both sides.

8. Place coated chicken breasts in the baking dish that you prepared.

9. Bake the chicken until it is tender and no longer pink in the center (you don't need to flip the chicken while baking). The baking should take about 25 to 30 minutes.

Cuban Black Beans and Rice

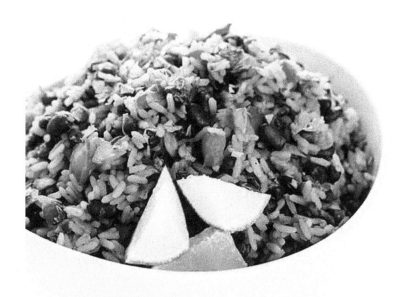

SmartPoints value: Green plan - 7SP, Blue plan - 4SP, Purple plan - 4SP

Total Time: 35 min, Prep time: 10 min, Cooking time: 25 min, Serves: 6

Nutritional value: Calories - 333.5, Carbs - 54.8g Fat - 5.1g, Protein - 16.1g

Ingredients

- Water - 2½ cup(s), divided
- Uncooked white rice (long grain-variety) - 1 cup(s)
- Olive oil - 2 tsp
- Banana pepper(s) - 1 medium
- Black beans (canned) - 31 oz, two 15.5 oz cans (undrained)
- Cilantro (fresh, chopped, divided) - ⅔ cup(s)
- Minced garlic - 1½ Tbsp
- Ground cumin - 1 tsp
- Uncooked red onion(s) (chopped) - 1¾ cup(s)
- Oregano (dried) - 1 tsp
- Table salt - 1 tsp (or to taste)
- Red wine vinegar - 1 Tbsp
- Lime(s) (fresh) - 1 medium, cut into six wedges

Instructions

1.   Bring two cups of water to a boil in a small saucepan and add the rice, then cook as package directs.

2.   Heat some oil in a large nonstick skillet over medium-high heat.

3.   Add a cup of chopped onions and all of the pepper, then cook, occasionally stirring, until it is tender; about 7 minutes.

4.   Toss in garlic, cumin, and oregano, then cook, stirring until fragrant; about 30 seconds.

5.   Stir in the beans and their liquid, the remaining half cup of water and salt, then bring to a simmer.

6.   Reduce the heat to low and simmer for the flavors to blend in about 5 minutes.

7.   Remove the dish from heat, then stir in vinegar and 1/3 cup of cilantro.

8.   To serve, use a spoon to put beans over rice and sprinkle it with 1/4 cup of the remaining onion and 1/3 cup of the remaining cilantro, then squeeze fresh lime juice over the top.

Note: If you desire, sprinkle the dish with salt before serving.

Spaghetti Squash With Fresh Tomato-Basil Sauce

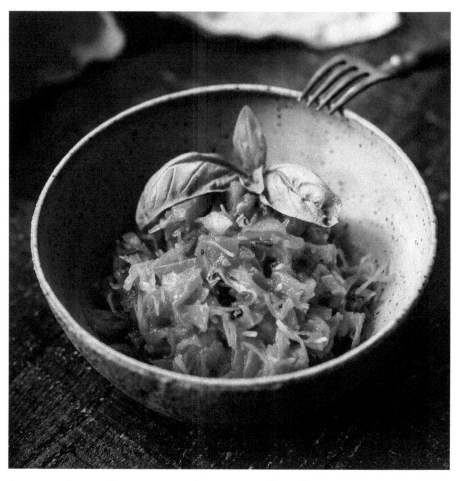

SmartPoints value: Green plan - 2SP, Blue plan - 2SP, Purple plan - 2SP

Total time: 30 min, Prep time: 15 min, Cooking time: 15 min, Serves: 4

Nutritional value: Calories - 216.2, Carbs - 14.2g Fat - 17.2g, Protein - 5.0g

Enjoy this recipe with its taste of summer. Ensure to cook it with very ripe tomatoes and fresh basil to get the best flavour.

Ingredients

- Tomato(es) (fresh) - 2¼ pound(s)
- Olive oil (extra virgin) - 2 Tbsp
- Minced garlic - 1¼ tsp, finely minced
- Basil (fresh, sliced) - ½ cup(s)
- Kosher salt - ½ tsp (or to taste)
- Black pepper (freshly ground) - ¼ tsp (or to taste)
- Spaghetti squash (uncooked) - 2½ pound(s)

Instructions

1.   Toss tomatoes, oil, garlic, basil, salt and pepper together in a large bowl and let it stand, occasionally tossing, until the tomatoes release their juices and the mixture is quite juicy; about 10 to 15 minutes.

2.   Cut the spaghetti squash in half and scoop out the seeds, then place the squash in a covered microwave-safe container.

3.   Cook the spaghetti squash on high power until strands of squash separate when you scrape the flesh with a fork; about 15 minutes. Alternatively, you can also roast the squash for about 20 minutes in the oven.

4. Scrape the spaghetti squash from the peel with a fork to form strands and add it to the bowl with tomatoes and toss to coat.

5. Notes: It would be delicious to add chunks of fresh mozzarella or freshly grated Parmesan cheese to this meal. However, it might affect the Smart Points value.

Barley, Grape Tomato And Arugula Sauté

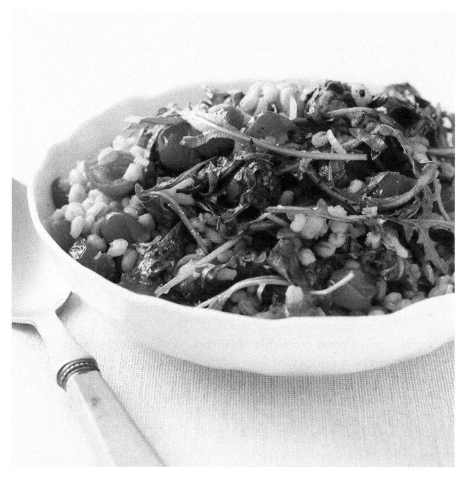

SmartPoints value: Green plan - 3SP, Blue plan - 3SP, Purple plan - 1SP

Total time: 50 min, Prep time: 10 min, Cooking time: 40 min, Serves: 4

Nutritional value: Calories - 82.8, Carbs - 4.8g Fat - 7.2g, Protein - 1.2g

This grain and vegetable side dish is colourful and sweet with a peppery bite.

Toss in some yellow grape tomatoes to add even more colour.

Ingredients

- Water - 1¼ cup(s)
- Table salt - ¾ tsp, divided
- Pearl barley (uncooked) - ½ cup(s)
- Olive oil (extra-virgin) - 1½ tsp, divided
- Tomatoes (grape) - 1½ cup(s), halved
- Minced garlic - 1½ tsp
- Black pepper (freshly ground) - ¼ tspArugula (baby leaves) - 3 cup(s)
- Lemon zest (finely grated) - ¼ tsp (or to taste)

Instructions

1.   Stir half tsp of salt into a small saucepan of water and bring it to a boil. Add barley to it and cover; reduce the heat to low and cook until the water is absorbed and the barley is tender but still has a nice bite to it; about 30-35 minutes. Remove the saucepan from the heat and set it aside.

2.   Apply heat to one teaspoon of oil in a medium nonstick skillet over medium-high heat. Add the tomatoes and garlic, then

sauté it until the tomatoes start to soften and release their juices; about 1-2 minutes.

3.   Put in more barley, the remaining one-quarter teaspoon of salt and pepper, and reduce the heat to medium and cook, stirring it until the tomatoes soften further and the grain absorbs tomato liquid; about 2-3 minutes.

4.   Stir in the arugula and toss it over medium heat until it wilts; about 30 seconds.

5.   Remove the dish from the heat and stir in the remaining half teaspoon of oil and lemon zest.

Note: You can reheat this recipe the next day, and it will still taste great. Alternatively, you can serve it as a cold salad. Allow it come to room temperature and then toss it, adding just a bit of red wine or balsamic vinegar.

Creamy Mushroom And Chicken Stew Crockpot

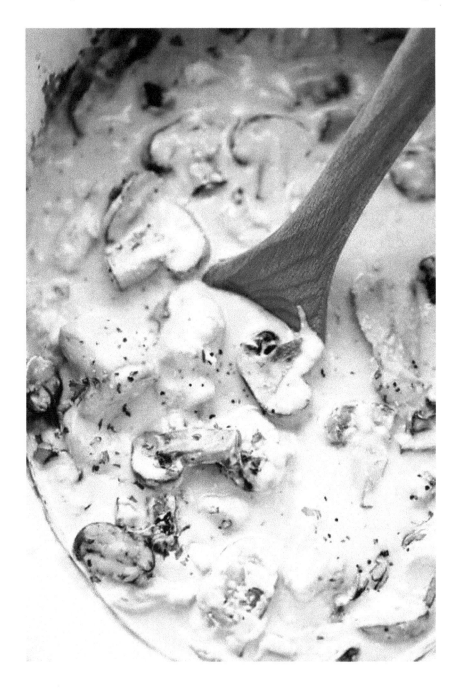

SmartPoints value: Green plan - 2SP, Blue plan - 2SP, Purple plan - 2SP

Total Time: 4hr 20min, Prep time: 10 min, Cooking time: 4hr 10mins,

Serves: 4

Nutritional value: Calories – 278, Carbs – 24.2g, Fat – 4.2g, Protein – 32g

The mushroom and chicken stew crockpot is a fantastic low-calorie dinner idea. It's a healthy and easy slow cooker recipe with great taste.

Ingredients

- Chicken breast (skinless) - 1 lb
- Baby portabella mushroom (sliced) - 8 oz
- Onion (finely chopped) - 1 piece
- Carrots (cut into matchsticks) - 1/2 cup
- Peas (fresh or frozen) - 1/2 cup
- Celery (chopped) - 2 stalks
- Mushroom seasoning (powdered) - 2 tbsp
- Chicken broth (fat-free) - 2 cups
- Sour cream (fat-free, at room temp) - 1 cup
- Garlic (minced) - 3 cloves

- Salt (1 tsp)

- Pepper (1/2 tsp)

Instructions

1. Combine all ingredients in a crockpot except the sour cream.

2. For 4- 6 hrs., cook on low heat.

3. For about 5 minutes, stir in sour cream, and warm until it is thoroughly heated. Serve immediately.

Smashed Avocado And Egg Toast

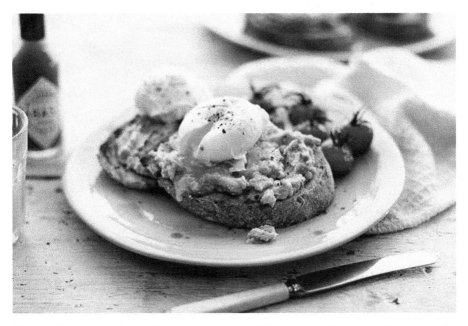

SmartPoints value: Green plan – 6SP, Blue plan – 4SP, Purple plan - 4SP

Total Time: 7 min, Prep time: 5 min, Cooking time: 2 min, Serves: 1

Nutritional value: Calories – 214.0, Carbs - 16.4g, Fat – 14.2g, Protein - 8.4g

Ingredients

- Avocado - ¼ item(s), medium-sized, ripe but still a touch firm

- Light whole-grain bread - 1 slice(s)

- Whole hard-boiled egg(s) - 1 item(s), sliced

- Table salt - 1 pinch

- Crushed red pepper flakes - 1 pinch

- Black pepper - 1 pinch

Instructions

1.   Place one slice of bread on a clean plate.

2.   Top with a portion of peeled avocado and gently smash with a knife or fork.

3.   Cut hard-boiled egg in half and place each half on the bread.

4.   Gently smash egg and mix with smashed avocado. Season the bread to taste with salt, pepper, and red pepper flakes.

5.   Cover with another slice of bread and place in a flat-sitting electric bread toaster.

6.   Remove smashed avocado and egg toast from the toaster once the "ready" light comes on.

Morning Porridge

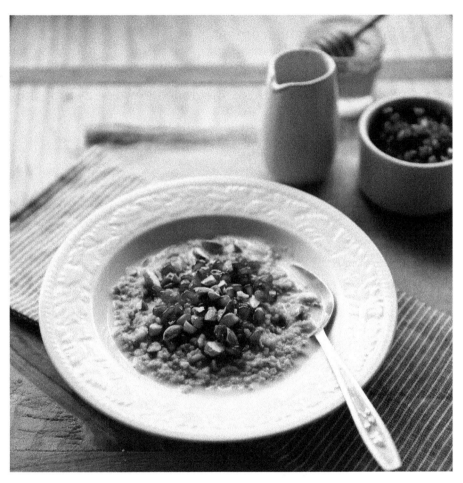

Serving: 2

Prep Time: 15 minutes

Cook Time: Nil

Ingredients:

- 2 tablespoons coconut flour
- 2 tablespoons vanilla protein powder
- 3 tablespoons Golden Flaxseed meal
- 1 ½ cups almond milk, unsweetened Powdered erythritol

How To:

1.   Take a bowl and blend in flaxseed meal, protein powder, coconut flour and blend well.

2.   Add mix to the saucepan (place over medium heat).

3.   Add almond milk and stir, let the mixture thicken .

4.   Add your required amount of sweetener and serve.

5.   Enjoy!

Nutrition (Per Serving)

Calories: 259

 Fat: 13g

Carbohydrates: 5g

Protein: 16g

Vanilla Sweet Potato Porridge

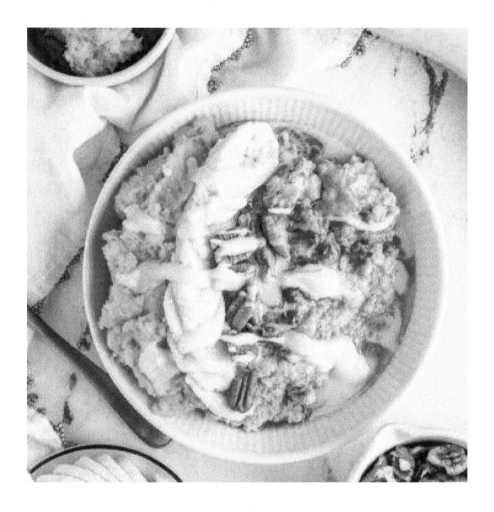

Serving: 5

Prep Time: 10 minutes

Cook Time: 8 hours

Ingredients:

- 6 sweet potatoes, peeled and cut into 1-inch cubes
- 1 ½ cups light coconut milk
- 1 teaspoon ground cinnamon
- 1 teaspoon ground cardamom
- 1 teaspoon pure vanilla extract
- 1 cup raisins Pinch of salt

How To:

1.　Add sweet potatoes coconut milk, vanilla, cardamom, cinnamon to your Slow Cooker.

2.　Close lid and cook on LOW for 8 hours.

3.　Open the lid and mash the entire mixture using potato masher to mash the sweet potatoes, stir well.

4.　Stir in raisins, salt and serve.

5.　Serve and enjoy!

Nutrition (Per Serving)

Calories: 317

Fat: 4g

Carbohydrates: 71g

Protein: 4g

A Nice German Oatmeal

Serving: 3

Prep Time: 10 minutes

Cook Time: 8 hours

Ingredients:

- 1 cup steel-cut oats
- 3 cups water
- 6 ounces coconut milk
- 2 tablespoons cocoa powder
- 1 tablespoon brown sugar
- 1 tablespoon coconut, shredded

How to
1. Grease the Slow Cooker well.
2. Add the listed ingredients to your Cooker and stir.
3. Place lid and cook on LOW for 8 hours.
4. Divide amongst serving bowls and enjoy!

Nutrition (Per Serving)

Calories: 200

Fat: 4g

Carbohydrates: 11g

Protein: 5g

Very Nutty Banana Oatmeal

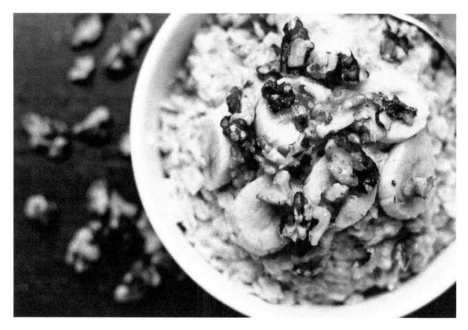

Serving: 4

Prep Time: 15 minutes

Cook Time: 7-9 hours

Ingredients:

- 1 cup steel-cut oats
- 1 ripe banana, mashed
- 2 cups unsweetened almond milk
- 1 cup water

- 1 ½ tablespoons honey
- ½ teaspoon vanilla extract
- ¼ cup almonds, chopped
- 1 teaspoon ground cinnamon
- ¼ teaspoon ground nutmeg

How To:

1. Grease the Slow Cooker well.
2. Add the listed ingredients to your Slow Cooker and stir.
3. Cover with lid and cook on LOW for 7-9 hours.
4. Serve and enjoy!

Nutrition (Per Serving)

Calories: 230

Fat: 7g

Carbohydrates: 40g

Protein: 5g

Black Bean Vegan Wraps

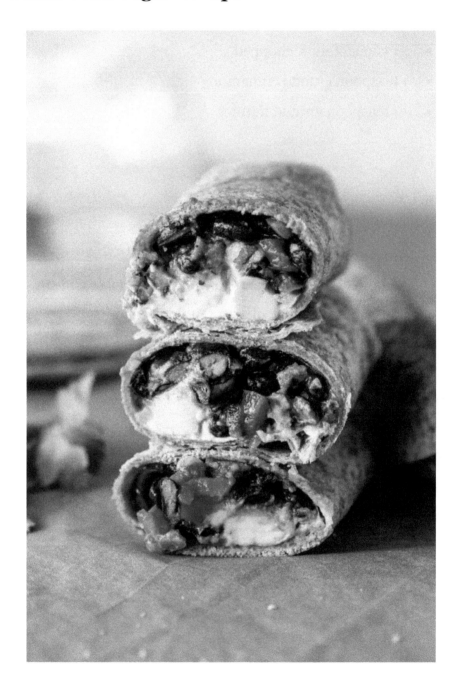

Nutritional Facts

servings per container   5

Prep Total   10 min

Serving Size 2/3 cup (27g)

Amount per serving 200

Calories

% Daily Value

Total Fat 8g 1%

Saturated Fat 1g   2%

Trans Fat 0g 2%

Cholesterol   2%

Sodium 240mg   7%

Total Carbohydrate 12g   2%

Dietary Fiber 4g   14%

Total Sugar 12g   01.21%

Protein 3g

Vitamin C 2mcg   2%

Calcium 20mg   1%

Iron 7mg   2%

Potassium 25mg   6%

Ingredients

- 1 1/2 half cup of beans (sprouted & cooked)
- 2 carrot
- 1 or 2 tomatoes
- 2 avocado
- 1 cob of corn
- 1 Kale
- 2 or 3 sticks of celery
  - 2 persimmons
- 1 Coriander

Dressing:

- 1 hachiyapersimmon (or half a mango)
- Juice of 1 lemon
- 2 to 3 tablespoons original olive oil
- 1/4 clean cup water
- 1 or 2 teaspoons grated fresh ginger
- 1/2 teaspoon of salt

Instructions:

1. Sprout & cook the black beans

2. Chop all the ingredients & mix them in a neat bowl with the black beans

3.   Mix all the ingredients for the dressing & pour into the salad

4.   Serve a spoonful in a clean lettuce leaf that you can easily roll into a wrap. Most people do use iceberg or romaine lettuce.

Fascinating Spinach and Beef Meatballs

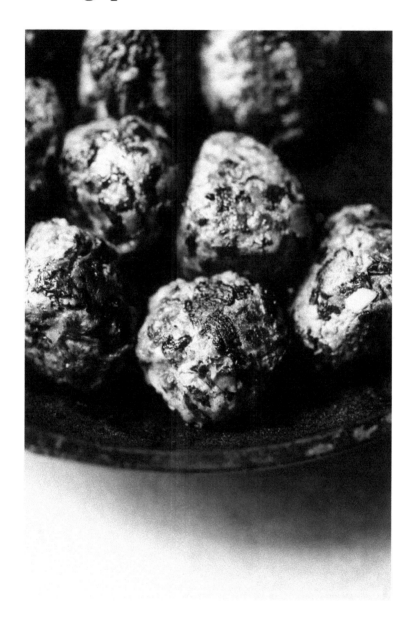

Serving: 4

Prep Time: 10 minutes

Cook Time: 20

Ingredients:

- ½ cup onion
- 4 garlic cloves
- 1 whole egg
- ¼ teaspoon oregano
- Pepper as needed
- 1 pound lean ground beef
- 10 ounces spinach

How To:

1. Preheat your oven to 375 degrees F.

2. Take a bowl and blend within the remainder of the ingredients, and using your hands, roll into meatballs.

3. Transfer to a sheet tray and bake for 20 minutes.

4. Enjoy!

Nutrition (Per Serving)

Calorie: 200

Fat: 8g

Carbohydrates: 5g

Protein: 29g

Juicy and Peppery Tenderloin

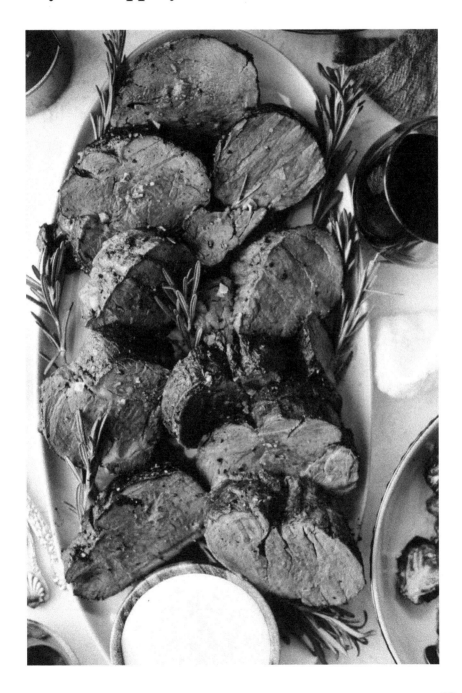

Serving: 4

Prep Time: 10 minutes

Cook Time: 20

Ingredients:

- 2 teaspoons sage, chopped
- Sunflower seeds and pepper
- 2 1/2 pounds beef tenderloin
- 2 teaspoons thyme, chopped
- 2 garlic cloves, sliced
- 2 teaspoons rosemary, chopped
- 4 teaspoons olive oil

How To:

1. Preheat your oven to 425 degrees F.

2. Take alittle knife and cut incisions within the tenderloin; insert one slice of garlic into the incision.

3. Rub meat with oil.

4. Take a bowl and add sunflower seeds, sage, thyme, rosemary, pepper and blend well.

5. Rub the spice mix over tenderloin.

6.   Put rubbed tenderloin into the roasting pan and bake for 10 minutes.

7.   Lower temperature to 350 degrees F and cook for 20 minutes more until an indoor thermometer reads 145 degrees F.

8.   Transfer tenderloin to a chopping board and let sit for 15 minutes; slice through 20 pieces and enjoy!

Nutrition (Per Serving)

Calorie: 183

Fat: 9g

Carbohydrates: 1g

Protein: 24g

Healthy Avocado Beef Patties

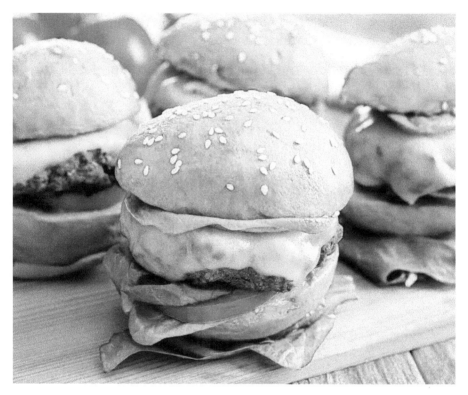

Serving: 2

Prep Time: 15 minutes

Cook Time: 10 minutes

Ingredients:

- 1 pound 85% lean ground beef

- 1 small avocado, pitted and peeled
- Fresh ground black pepper as needed

How To:

1. Pre-heat and prepare your broiler to high.
2. Divide beef into two equal-sized patties.
3. Season the patties with pepper accordingly.
4. Broil the patties for five minutes per side.
5. Transfer the patties to a platter.
6. Slice avocado into strips and place them on top of the patties.

7. Serve and enjoy!

Nutrition (Per Serving)

Calories: 568

Fat: 43g

Net Carbohydrates: 9g

Protein: 38g

Ravaging Beef Pot Roast

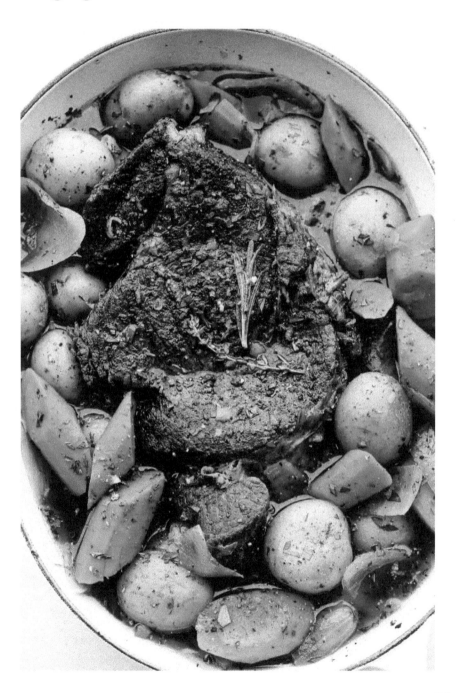

Serving: 4

Prep Time: 10 minutes

Cook Time: 75 minutes

Ingredients:

- 3 ½ pounds beef roast
- 4 ounces mushrooms, sliced
- 12 ounces beef stock
- 1-ounce onion soup mix
- ½ cup Italian dressing, low sodium, and low fat

How To:

1.   Take a bowl and add the stock, onion soup mix and Italian dressing
2.   Stir.
3.   Put roast beef in pan.
4.   Add mushrooms, stock mix to the pan and canopy with foil.
5.   Preheat your oven to 300 degrees F.
6.   Bake for 1 hour and quarter-hour .
7.   Let the roast cool.

8. Slice and serve.

9. Enjoy with the gravy on top!

Nutrition (Per Serving)

Calories: 700

Fat: 56g

Carbohydrates: 10g

Protein: 70g

Lettuce and Chicken Platter

Serving: 6

Prep Time: 10 minutes

Cook Time: nil

Ingredients:

- 2 cups chicken, cooked and coarsely chopped ½ head ice berg lettuce, sliced and chopped 1 celery rib, chopped
- 1 medium apple, cut
- ½ red bell pepper, deseeded and chopped 6-7 green olives, pitted and halved 1 red onion, chopped

For dressing
- 1 tablespoon raw honey
- 2 tablespoons lemon juice
- Salt and pepper to taste

How To:

1. Cut the vegetables and transfer them to your Salad Bowl.
2. Add olives.

3.   Chop the cooked chicken and transfer to your Salad bowl.

4.   Prepare dressing by mixing the ingredients listed under

Dressing.

5.   Pour the dressing into the Salad bowl.

6.   Toss and enjoy!

Nutrition (Per Serving)

Calories: 296

Fat: 21g

Carbohydrates: 9g

Protein: 18g

Greek Lemon Chicken Bowl

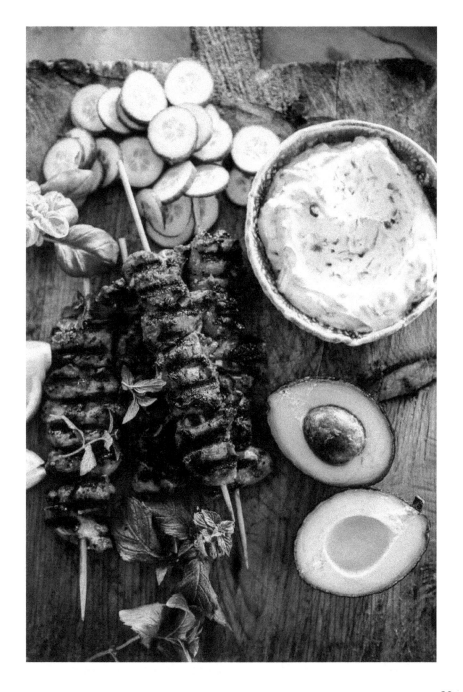

Serving: 6

Prep Time: 10 minutes

Cook Time: 15 minutes

Ingredients:

- 2 cups chicken, cooked and chopped
- 2 cans chicken broth, fat free
- 2 medium carrots, chopped
- ¼ teaspoon pepper
- 2 tablespoons parsley, snipped
- ¼ cup lemon juice
- 1 can cream chicken soup, fat free, low sodium ½ cup onion, chopped
- 1 garlic clove, minced

How To:

1. Take a pot and add all the ingredients except parsley into it.
2. Season with salt and pepper.
3. Bring the combination to a overboil medium-high heat.
4. Reduce the warmth and simmer for quarter-hour .

5.   Garnish with parsley.

6.   Serve hot and enjoy!

Nutrition (Per Serving)

Calories: 520

Fat: 33g

Carbohydrates: 31g

Protein: 30g

Chilled Chicken, Artichoke and Zucchini Platter

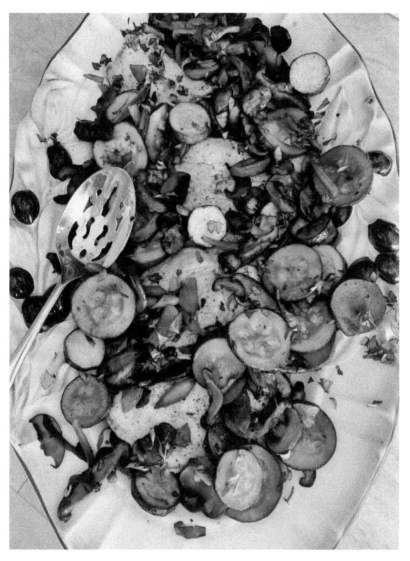

Serving: 4

Prep Time: 10 minutes

Cook Time: 5 minutes

Ingredients:

- 2 medium chicken breasts, cooked and cut into 1-inch cubes ¼ cup extra virgin olive oil
- 2 cups artichoke hearts, drained and roughly chopped
- 3 large zucchini, diced/cut into small rounds
- 1 can (15 ounce) chickpeas
- 1 cup Kalamata olives
- ½ teaspoon Fresh ground black pepper
- ½ teaspoon Italian seasoning
- ¼ cup parmesan, grated

How To:

1.   Take an outsized skillet and place it over medium heat, heat up vegetable oil .

2.   Add zucchini and sauté for five minutes, season with salt and pepper.

3.   Remove from heat and add all the listed ingredients to the skillet.

4.   Stir until combined.

5.   Transfer to glass container and store.

6.   Serve and enjoy!

Nutrition (Per Serving)

Calories: 457

Fat: 22g

Carbohydrates: 30g

Protein: 24g

Chicken and Carrot Stew

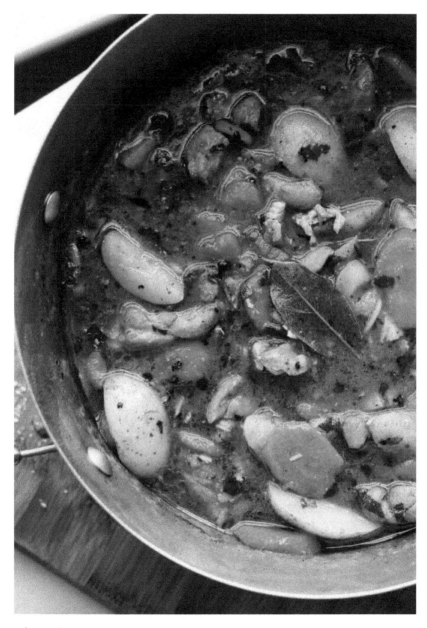

Serving: 6

Prep Time: 15 minutes

Cook Time: 6 hours

Ingredients:

- 4 chicken breasts, boneless and cubed
- 2 cups chicken broth
- 1 cup tomatoes, chopped
- 3 cups carrots, peeled and cubed
- 1 teaspoon thyme dried
- 1 cup onion, chopped
- 2 garlic clove, minced
- Pepper to taste

How To:

1. Add all the ingredients to the Slow Cooker.
2. Stir and shut the lid.
3. Cook for six hours.
4. Serve hot and enjoy!

Nutrition (Per Serving)

Calories: 182

Fat: 4g

Carbohydrates: 10g

Protein: 39g

Tasty Spinach Pie

Serving: 2

Prep Time: 10 minutes

Cooking Time: 4 hours

Ingredients:

- 10 ounces spinach
- 2 cups baby Bella mushrooms, chopped
- 1 red bell pepper, chopped
- 1 ½ cups low-fat cheese, shredded
- 8 whole eggs
- 1 cup coconut cream
- 2 tablespoons chives, chopped
- Pinch of pepper
- ½ cup almond flour
- ¼ teaspoon baking soda

How To:

1.   Take a bowl and add eggs, coconut milk , chives, pepper and whisk well.

2.   Add almond flour, bicarbonate of soda , cheese, mushrooms bell pepper, spinach and toss well.

3.   Grease your cooker and transfer mix to the Slow Cooker.

4.   Place lid and cook on LOW for 4 hours.

5.   Slice and enjoy!

Nutrition (Per Serving)

Calories: 201

Fat: 6g

Carbohydrates: 8g

Protein: 5g

Caramelized Banana & Blueberry Tacos

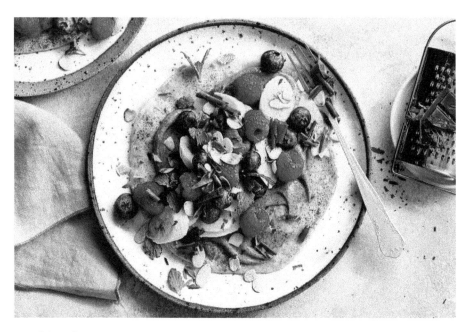

Nutritional Facts

servings per container   7

Prep Total   10 min

Serving Size 2/3 cup (51g)

Amount per serving
11
Calories

            % Daily Value

Total Fat 2g   2%

Saturated Fat 7g   10%

Trans Fat 3g 8%

Cholesterol   9%

Sodium 470mg   2%

Total Carbohydrate 20g   200%

Dietary Fiber 10g   20%

Total Sugar 9g   1%

Protein 6g

Vitamin C 1mcg   20%

Calcium 700mg   7%

Iron 7mg   2%

Potassium 470mg   9%

Ingredients

- 4 flour tortillas
- 1 Teaspoon coconut oil
- 2 ripe bananas, peeled and sliced lengthways into 0.5cm / 0.2" slices
- 100g / 3.5oz fresh blueberries

- 1 Teaspoon maple syrup
- 3 Teaspoon vanilla favored coconut or soy yogurt

- 1 heaped teaspoon tahini

- 1.5 Teaspoon shredded coconut or coconut flakes

- 1 Teaspoon cacao nibs

Instructions:

1. You will need to preheat the oven to 160°C / 320°F.

2. Kindly wrap the tortillas in foil & heat in the oven for 6 minutes.

3. Heat a medium-sized, heavy-based, non-stick or cast-iron skillet on medium heat on the stove. Add original coconut oil & once it's melted, add the sliced clean bananas.

4. Fry the bananas until they are golden brown on both sides, making sure to rotate them frequently so they won't stick to the pan.

5. You need to top the warm tortillas with the fried bananas and drizzle with tahini, yogurt, and maple syrup.

6. Kindly top with blueberries and sprinkle with coconut and cacao nibs.

7. Serve and enjoy

Decent Beef and Onion Stew

Serving: 4

Prep Time: 10 minutes

Cook Time 1-2 hours

Ingredients:

- 2 pounds lean beef, cubed
- 3 pounds shallots, peeled
- 5 garlic cloves, peeled, whole
- 3 tablespoons tomato paste
- 1 bay leaves
- ¼ cup olive oil
- 3 tablespoons lemon juice

How To:

1. Take a stew pot and place it over medium heat.
2. Add vegetable oil and let it heat up.
3. Add meat and brown.
4. Add remaining ingredients and canopy with water.

5. Bring the entire mix to a boil.

6. Reduce heat to low and canopy the pot.

7. Simmer for 1-2 hours until beef is cooked thoroughly.

8. Serve hot!

Nutrition (Per Serving)

Calories: 136

Fat: 3g

Carbohydrates: 0.9g

Protein: 24g

Clean Parsley and Chicken Breast

Serving: 2

Prep Time: 10 minutes

Cook Time: 40 minutes

Ingredients:

- 1/2 tablespoon dry parsley
- 1/2 tablespoon dry basil
- 2 chicken breast halves, boneless and skinless 1/4 teaspoon sunflower seeds
- 1/4 teaspoon red pepper flakes, crushed 1 tomato, sliced

How To:

1. Pre-heat your oven to 350 degrees F.

2. Take a 9x13 inch baking dish and grease it up with cooking spray.

3. Sprinkle 1 tablespoon of parsley, 1 teaspoon of basil and spread the mixture over your baking dish.

4. Arrange the pigeon breast halves over the dish and sprinkle garlic slices on top.

5.	Take a little bowl and add 1 teaspoon parsley, 1 teaspoon of basil, sunflower seeds, basil, red pepper and blend well. Pour the mixture over the pigeon breast .

6.	Top with tomato slices and canopy , bake for 25 minutes.

7.	Remove the duvet and bake for quarter-hour more.

8.	Serve and enjoy!

Nutrition (Per Serving)

Calories: 150

Fat: 4g

Carbohydrates: 4g

Protein: 25g

Zucchini Beef Sauté with Coriander Greens

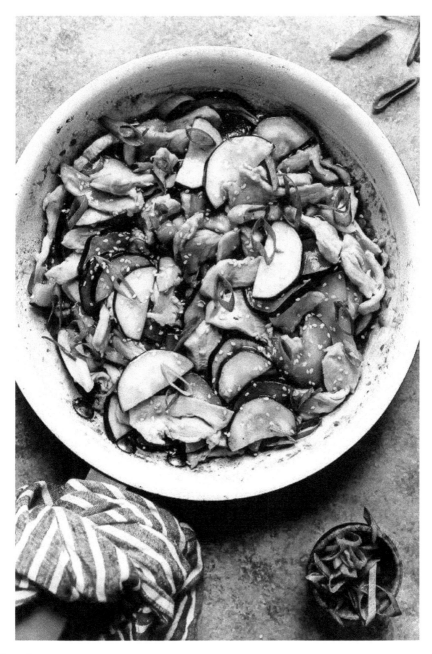

Serving: 4

Prep Time: 10 minutes

Cook Time: 10 minutes

Ingredients:

- 10 ounces beef, sliced into 1-2-inch strips
- 1 zucchini, cut into 2-inch strips
- ¼ cup parsley, chopped
- 3 garlic cloves, minced
- 2 tablespoons tamari sauce
- 4 tablespoons avocado oil

How To:

1.   Add 2 tablespoons avocado oil during a frypan over high heat.

2.   Place strips of beef and brown for a couple of minutes on high heat.

3.   Once the meat is brown, add zucchini strips and sauté until tender.

4.   Once tender, add tamari sauce, garlic, parsley and allow them to sit for a couple of minutes more.

5.   Serve immediately and enjoy!

Nutrition (Per Serving)

Calories: 500

Fat: 40g

Carbohydrates: 5g

Protein: 31g

Hearty Lemon and Pepper Chicken

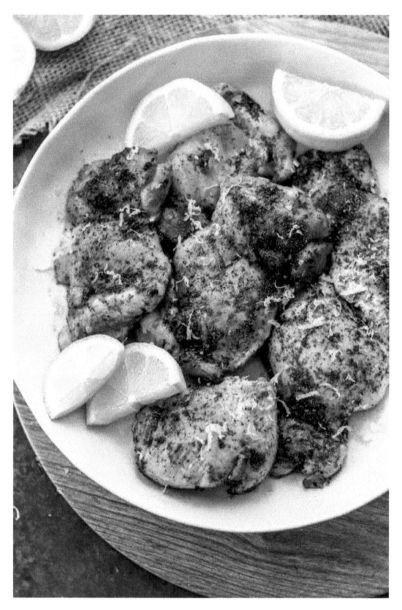

Serving: 4

Prep Time: 5 minutes

Cook Time: 15

Ingredients:

- 2 teaspoons olive oil
- 1 ¼ pounds skinless chicken cutlets
- 2 whole eggs
- ¼ cup panko crumbs
- 1 tablespoon lemon pepper
- Sunflower seeds and pepper to taste
- 3 cups green beans
- ¼ cup parmesan cheese
- ¼ teaspoon garlic powder

How To:

1. Pre-heat your oven to 425 degrees F.

2. Take a bowl and stir in seasoning, parmesan, lemon pepper, garlic powder, panko.

3. Whisk eggs in another bowl.

4. Coat cutlets in eggs and press into panko mix.

5.   Transfer coated chicken to a parchment lined baking sheet.

6.   Toss the beans in oil, pepper, add sunflower seeds, and lay them on the side of the baking sheet.

7.   Bake for quarter-hour .

8.   Enjoy!

Nutrition (Per Serving)

Calorie: 299

Fat: 10g

Carbohydrates: 10g

Protein: 43g

Sweet and Sour Cabbage and Apples

Serving: 4

Prep Time: 15 minutes

Cook Time: 8 hours

Ingredients:

- ¼ cup honey
- ¼ cup apple cider vinegar
- 2 tablespoons Orange Chili-Garlic Sauce
- 1 teaspoon sea salt
- 3 sweet tart apples, peeled, cored and sliced
- 2 heads green cabbage, cored and shredded
- 1 sweet red onion, thinly sliced

How To:

1.   Take alittle bowl and whisk in honey, orange-chili aioli , vinegar.

2.   Stir well.

3.   Add honey mix, apples, onion and cabbage to your Slow Cooker and stir.

4.   Close lid and cook on LOW for 8 hours.

5.   Serve and enjoy!

Nutrition (Per Serving)

Calories: 164

Fat: 1g

Carbohydrates: 41g

Protein: 4g

Delicious Aloo Palak

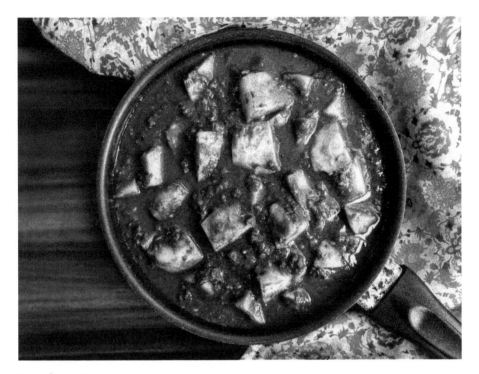

Serving: 6

Prep Time: 10 minutes

Cook Time: 6-8 hours

Ingredients:

- 2 pounds red potatoes, chopped
- 1 small onion, diced

- 1 red bell pepper, seeded and diced
- ¼ cup fresh cilantro, chopped
- 1/3 cup low-sodium veggie broth
- 1 teaspoon salt
- ½ teaspoon Garam masala
- ½ teaspoon ground cumin
- ¼ teaspoon ground turmeric
- ¼ teaspoon ground coriander
- ¼ teaspoon freshly ground black pepper 2 pounds fresh spinach, chopped

How To:

1.   Add potatoes, bell pepper, onion, cilantro, broth and seasoning to your Slow Cooker.

2.   Mix well.

3.   Add spinach on top.

4.   Place lid and cook on LOW for 6-8 hours.

5.   Stir and serve.

6.   Enjoy!

Nutrition (Per Serving)

Calories: 205

Fat: 1g

Carbohydrates: 44g

Protein: 9g

Orange and Chili Garlic Sauce

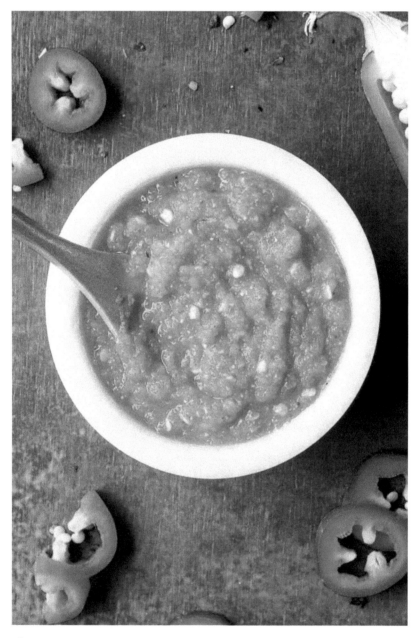

Serving: 5 cups

Prep Time: 15 minutes

Cook Time: 8 hours

Ingredients:

- ½ cup apple cider vinegar
- 4 pounds red jalapeno peppers, stems, seeds and ribs removed, chopped
- 10 garlic cloves, chopped
- ½ cup tomato paste
- Juice of 1 orange zest
- ½ cup honey
- 2 tablespoons soy sauce
- 2 teaspoons salt

How To:

1. Add vinegar, garlic, peppers, ingredient , fruit juice , honey, zest, soy and salt to your Slow Cooker.

2. Stir and shut lid.

3. Cook on LOW for 8 hours.

4. Use as required !

Nutrition (Per Serving)

Calories: 33

Fat: 1g

Carbohydrates: 8g

Protein: 1g

Tantalizing Mushroom Gravy

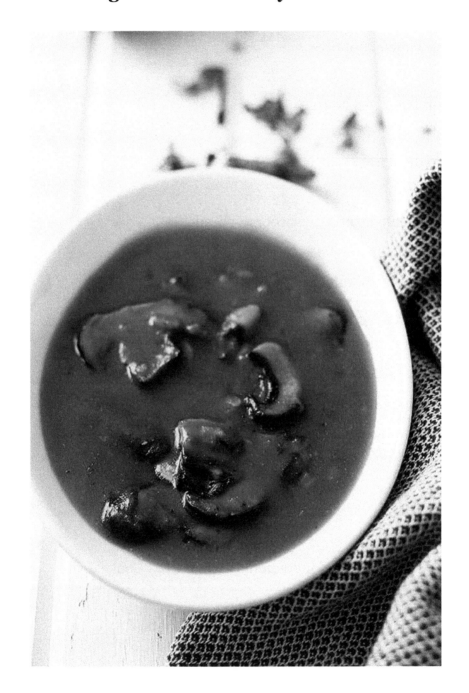

Serving: 2 cups

Prep Time: 5 minutes

Cook Time: 5-8 hours

Ingredients:

- 1 cup button mushrooms, sliced
- ¾ cup low-fat buttermilk
- 1/3 cup water
- 1 medium onion, finely diced
- 2 garlic cloves, minced
- 2 tablespoons extra virgin olive oil
- 2 tablespoons all-purpose flour
- 1 tablespoon fresh rosemary, minced Freshly ground black pepper

How To:

1. Add the listed ingredients to your Slow Cooker.

2. Place lid and cook on LOW for 5-8 hours.

3. Serve warm and use as needed!

Nutrition (Per Serving)

Calories: 54

Fat: 4g

Carbohydrates: 4g

Protein: 2g

Everyday Vegetable Stock

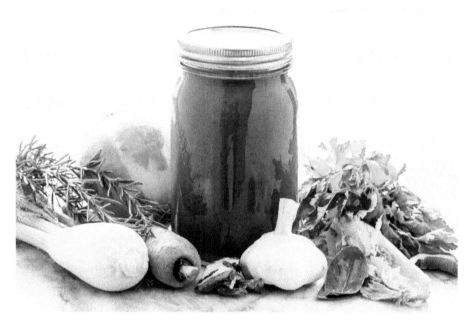

Serving: 10 cups

Prep Time: 5 minutes

Cook Time: 8-12 hours

Ingredients:

- 2 celery stalks (with leaves), quartered

- 4 ounces mushrooms, with stems

- 2 carrots, unpeeled and quartered

- 1 onion, unpeeled, quartered from pole to pole

- 1 garlic head, unpeeled, halved across middle
- 2 fresh thyme sprigs
- 10 peppercorns
- ½ teaspoon salt
- Enough water to fill 3 quarters of Slow Cooker

How To:

1.   Add celery, mushrooms, onion, carrots, garlic, thyme, salt, peppercorn and water to your Slow Cooker.

2.   Stir and canopy .

3.   Cook on LOW for 8-12 hours.

4.   Strain the stock through a fine mesh cloth/metal mesh and discard solids.

5.   Use as needed.

Nutrition (Per Serving)

Calories: 38

Fat: 5g

Carbohydrates: 1g

Protein: 0g

Creamy Cauliflower Pakora Soup

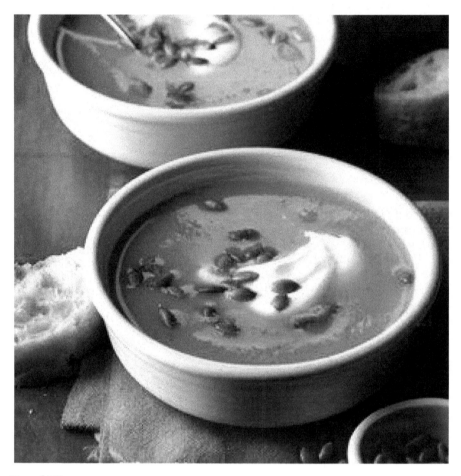

Total Time

Prep: 20 min. Cook: 20 min.

Makes

8 servings (3 quarts)

Ingredients:

- 1 huge head cauliflower, cut into little florets
- 5 medium potatoes, stripped and diced
- 1 huge onion, diced
- 4 medium carrots, stripped and diced
- 2 celery ribs, diced
- 1 container (32 ounces) vegetable stock
- 1 teaspoon garam masala
- 1 teaspoon garlic powder
- 1 teaspoon ground coriander
- 1 teaspoon ground turmeric
- 1 teaspoon ground cumin
- 1 teaspoon pepper
- 1 teaspoon salt
- 1/2 teaspoon squashed red pepper chips
- Water or extra vegetable stock New cilantro leaves
- Lime wedges, discretionary

Directions

1. In a Dutch stove over medium-high warmth, heat initial 14 fixings to the point of boiling. Cook and mix until vegetables are

delicate, around 20 minutes. Expel from heat; cool marginally. Procedure in groups in a blender or nourishment processor until smooth. Modify consistency as wanted with water (or extra stock). Sprinkle with new cilantro. Serve hot, with lime wedges whenever wanted.

2.   Stop alternative: Before including cilantro, solidify cooled soup in cooler compartments. To utilize, in part defrost in cooler medium-term. Warmth through in a pan, blending every so often and including a little water if fundamental. Sprinkle with cilantro. Whenever wanted, present with lime wedges.